Nursing & Health Survival Guide

T0186314

2nd Edition

Kerry Reid-Searl
Trudy Dwyer
Lorna Moxham
Jo Reid-Speirs
Ann Richards

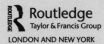

Routledge
Taylor & Francis Group

LONDON AND NEW YORK

First published 2012 by Pearson Education Limited

Published 2014 by Routledge
2 Park Square, Milton Park, Abingdon, Oxon OX14 4RN
711 Third Avenue, New York, NY 10017, USA

Routledge is an imprint of the Taylor & Francis Group, an informa business

Copyright © 2012, Taylor & Francis.

The rights of Kerry Reid-Searl, Trudy Dwyer, Lorna Moxham, Jo Reid-Speirs and
Ann Richards to be identified as authors of this Work has been asserted by them
in accordance, with the Copyright, Designs and Patents Act 1988.

Notices
Knowledge and best practice in this field are constantly changing. As new research and expe
broaden our understanding, changes in research methods, professional practices, or medica
treatment may become necessary.

Practitioners and researchers must always rely on their own experience and knowledge in
evaluating and using any information, methods, compounds, or experiments described herein
using such information or methods they should be mindful of their own safety and the safety
others, including parties for whom they have a professional responsibility.

To the fullest extent of the law, neither the Publisher nor the authors, contributors, or editors,
assume any liability for any injury and/or damage to persons or property as a matter of produ
liability, negligence or otherwise, or from any use or operation of any methods, products,
instructions, or ideas contained in the material herein.

ISBN 13: 978-0-273-76446-5 (hbk)

British Library Cataloguing-in-Publication Data
A catalogue record for this book is available from the British Library

Library of Congress Cataloging-in-Publication Data
A catalog record for this book is available from the Library of Congress

Typeset in 8/9.5pt Helvetica by 35

contents

All nurses need an understanding of maths. Correct and safe administration of medication depends upon the nurse's ability to both calculate and measure medications correctly.

This book has been designed as a quick reference to assist you in medication administration. It is not intended to be a replacement for more comprehensive mathematical books that can guide you further.

The book is designed to provide prompts and guidelines pertaining to information necessary to administer medications safely. It does this by:

- Revisiting some basic mathematical manipulations.
- Giving you some useful information that can help you to consider whether your dosages are reasonable.
- Providing you with a reference to standard formulas.
- Revisiting essential information in terms of safe medication administration.

When working out dosages of what you are required to administer, the following approach should be used:

- Read the medication order/prescription thoroughly.
- Read the medication drug packaging.
- Sort out what the dosage problem is.
- Use your mathematical manipulation skills to convert measuring units if necessary.
- Apply the appropriate formula and calculate.

- Reflect on the dosage:
  - a Is this reasonable?
  - b Is this within normal range?
  - c What are the consequences to the patient with this dosage?
- Check the dosage and your calculations.

Maths revisited

■ MATHEMATICAL SYMBOLS

TERMINOLOGY	SYMBOL
Equal to	=
Not equal to	≠
Approximately equal to	≈
Greater than	>
Less than	<
Square root	√
Per cent	%
Degree	°
Ratio	:

■ ORDER OF OPERATIONS

There are four fundamental operations used to solve
mathematical problems. These are:

1. Addition   +
2. Subtraction   −
3. Multiplication   ×
4. Division   ÷

If a mathematical problem requires more than one operation, there is a rule of order for performing each operation. This is best remembered as **BIDMAS** (the mnemonic 'Belly Itches Do Make A Scratch').

1st	Brackets	( )
2nd	Index notation	4^3 or 'to the power of'
3rd	Division	$\div$
4th	Multiplication	$\times$
5th	Addition	$+$
6th	Subtraction	$-$

Step 1 Work out all the sums in the brackets.
Step 2 Do Index notation or 'to the power of'.
Step 3 Do $\div$ or $\times$ working from left to right, whichever comes first.
Step 4 Do $+$ or $-$ working from left to right, whichever comes first.

$$\begin{array}{cccc} \text{2nd} & \text{1st} & \text{4th} & \text{3rd} \\ \downarrow & \downarrow & \downarrow & \downarrow \end{array}$$

Rule applied: $70 \div (2 + 3) - 2 \times 2 = 10$ (✓)
Rule not applied: $70 \div (2 + 3) - 2 \times 2 = 72$ (✗)

■ NUMBER FACT GRIDS

Below is an **addition** grid for quick reference with basic addition facts up to 20.

+	1	2	3	4	5	6	7	8	9	10
1	2	3	4	5	6	7	8	9	10	11
2	3	4	5	6	7	8	9	10	11	12
3	4	5	6	7	8	9	10	11	12	13
4	5	6	7	8	9	10	11	12	13	14
5	6	7	8	9	10	11	12	13	14	15
6	7	8	9	10	11	12	13	14	15	16
7	8	9	10	11	12	13	14	15	16	17
8	9	10	11	12	13	14	15	16	17	18
9	10	11	12	13	14	15	16	17	18	19
10	11	12	13	14	15	16	17	18	19	20

The **multiplication** grid is a useful tool for quick reference of multiplication tables up to 12×.

×	1	2	3	4	5	6	7	8	9	10	11	12
1	1	2	3	4	5	6	7	8	9	10	11	12
2	2	4	6	8	10	12	14	16	18	20	22	24
3	3	6	9	12	15	18	21	24	27	30	33	36
4	4	8	12	16	20	24	28	32	36	40	44	48
5	5	10	15	20	25	30	35	40	45	50	55	60
6	6	12	18	24	30	36	42	48	54	60	66	72
7	7	14	21	28	35	42	49	56	63	70	77	84
8	8	16	24	32	40	48	56	64	72	80	88	96
9	9	18	27	36	45	54	63	72	81	90	99	108
10	10	20	30	40	50	60	70	80	90	100	110	120
11	11	22	33	44	55	66	77	88	99	110	121	132
12	12	24	36	48	60	72	84	96	108	120	132	144

■ TIME

Time is one of the five rights of medication administration.

All medication charts should have drug times written in 24-hour time.

For this reason nurses must be familiar with time and the 24-hour clock.

Units of time and conversions

1 minute (min)	60 seconds (s)	52 weeks	1 year (y)
1 hour (h)	60 minutes	365 days	1 year
1 day (d)	24 hours	366 days	1 leap year
1 week (w)	7 days	12 months	1 year
2 weeks	1 fortnight	10 years	1 decade
4 weeks	1 month (mth)	100 years	1 century

24-hour time

0000	00:00 midnight
0100	1:00 a.m.
0200	2:00 a.m.
0300	3:00 a.m.
0400	4:00 a.m.
0500	5:00 a.m.
0600	6:00 a.m.
0700	7:00 a.m.
0800	8:00 a.m.

0900	9:00 a.m.
1000	10:00 a.m.
1100	11:00 a.m.
1200	12:00 midday
1300	1:00 p.m.
1400	2:00 p.m.
1500	3:00 p.m.
1600	4:00 p.m.
1700	5:00 p.m.
1800	6:00 p.m.
1900	7:00 p.m.
2000	8:00 p.m.
2100	9:00 p.m.
2200	10:00 p.m.
2300	11:00 p.m.

■ HINDU-ARABIC AND ROMAN NUMERALS

HINDU-ARABIC	ROMAN
0	
1	I
2	II
3	III
4	IV

HINDU-ARABIC	ROMAN
5	V
6	VI
7	VII
8	VIII
9	IX
10	X
20	XX
30	XXX
40	XL
50	L
60	LX
70	LXX
80	LXXX
90	XC
100	C
500	D
1 000	M
10 000	X̄

■ FRACTION, DECIMAL AND PERCENTAGE CONVERSIONS

In medication administration, nurses are required to have an understanding of fractions, decimals and percentages. The following is a quick reference guide for simple conversions.

FRACTION	SIMPLIFIED FRACTION	TERMINOLOGY	DECIMAL FRACTION	PERCENTAGE
$\dfrac{10}{100}$	$\dfrac{1}{10}$	One-tenth	0.1 (0.10)	10%
$\dfrac{20}{100}$	$\dfrac{1}{5}$	One-fifth	0.2 (0.20)	20%
$\dfrac{25}{100}$	$\dfrac{1}{4}$	One-quarter	0.25	25%
$\dfrac{30}{100}$	$\dfrac{3}{10}$	Three-tenths	0.3 (0.30)	30%
$\dfrac{33}{100}$	$\dfrac{1}{3}$	One-third	0.33	33%
$\dfrac{40}{100}$	$\dfrac{2}{5}$	Two-fifths	0.4 (0.40)	40%

FRACTION	SIMPLIFIED FRACTION	TERMINOLOGY	DECIMAL FRACTION	PERCENTAGE
$\dfrac{50}{100}$	$\dfrac{1}{2}$	One-half	0.5 (0.50)	50%
$\dfrac{60}{100}$	$\dfrac{3}{5}$	Three-fifths	0.6 (0.60)	60%
$\dfrac{66}{100}$	$\dfrac{2}{3}$	Two-thirds	0.66	66%
$\dfrac{70}{100}$	$\dfrac{7}{10}$	Seven-tenths	0.7 (0.70)	70%
$\dfrac{75}{100}$	$\dfrac{3}{4}$	Three-quarters	0.75	75%
$\dfrac{80}{100}$	$\dfrac{4}{5}$	Four-fifths	0.8 (0.80)	80%

■ THE BASE SYSTEM

The base 10 (ten) system uses the digits 0, 1, 2, 3, 4, 5, 6, 7, 8, 9. The decimal system is an example of a base 10 system. Each of the digits has a face value and a place value. Place value is important in the decimal system and is fundamental to drug administration. In the base 10 system each place has a value 10 times that of the place value to the right of it, and one-tenth of the place value to the left. For example, 10 is ten times greater than 1, and ten times less than 100.

The place-value chart below indicates placement value. Numbers to the **left** side of the **decimal point** are greater than one, numbers to the **right** of the decimal point are less than one and represent fractions.

Place-value chart

PLACE VALUE	MILLION 1 000 000	HUNDRED THOUSANDS 100 000	TEN THOUSANDS 10 000	THOUSANDS 1 000
Exponential notation	10^6	10^5	10^4	10^3

Decimal Point
↓

HUNDREDS 100	TENS 10	ONES 1	•	TENTHS 1/10	HUNDREDTHS 1/100	THOUSANDTHS 1/1000
10^2	10^1			0.10	0.01	0.001

Reference / Adapted from Glaister, K. (1997) *Medication Mathematics*, *Melbourne*: Macmillan Education Australia, pp. 2 and 3.

■ THE DECIMAL POINT

In medication administration, errors can occur when calculating dosages if observation of the decimal point placement is not adhered to.

IMPORTANT RULE: DECIMALS AND DRUG ADMINISTRATION

When working with decimal fractions always place a zero to the left of the decimal point to indicate there are no whole numbers. Importantly, *do not* add a zero after a decimal point when working with a whole number.

Example

Use **0.34** if the dose is **.34**
If the dose was written as .34 it could be mistaken as 34.
Adding a zero to a whole number could also cause a mistake.

Example

If the dose was calculated to be **3. mg** do not add a zero after the decimal point to the whole number as this could be read as **30 mg**.

■ MEASURING A FLUID BALANCE CHART

If a patient is on a 24-hour fluid balance restriction, the nurse should be able to determine the volume per hour that the patient is allowed, and also determine if the patient has a positive or negative balance. In adding and subtracting volumes working with decimals may be required.

TIME	ORAL/NGT	VOL (mL)	INTRAVENOUS FLUID	VOL. (mL)	URINE (mL)	NGT ASPIRATE (mL)	VOMIT (mL)	FAECES	COMMENT
0800	Water	10	0.9% N/Saline (1000 mL)						
0900			N/Saline	84	150		30		
1000			N/Saline	84					
1100	Tea	100	N/Saline	84					
1200	Soup	100	N/Saline	84	240				
1300			N/Saline	84					
1400					150				
1500									
1600									
1700									
1800	Soup	200							
1900	Tea	250							
2000					250				
2100									

TIME	ORAL/ NGT	VOL (mL)	INTRAVENOUS FLUID	VOL (mL)	URINE (mL)	NGT ASPIRATE (mL)	VOMIT (mL)	FAECES	COMMENT
2300									
0000									
0100									
0200									
0300					300				
0400									
0500	Milk	200							
0600	Tea	250							
0700					250				
24-hour total		1110		420	1340		30		

Total intake (mL) 1530   Total output (mL) 1370

Source: Table on pages 14–15: **Reference** / Rockhampton Hospital, Queensland Health (1998) 24-Hour Fluid Balance Chart, June 1998. Brisbane: Queensland Health. Reproduced with permission.

The patient has a greater intake than output. Therefore the patient has a positive balance of 160 mL. 1530 – 1370 = 160

■ REVISITING BASIC ALGORITHMS

Vertical addition

HINTS

- Always apply the 'PUP' (points under points) rule when adding decimals.
- Addition is carried out moving in columns from right to left. ←
- The answer to addition of **two numbers** can be easily checked by applying an inverse or reverse operation of subtraction, i.e. subtract one number from the answer and the other number should remain.

PROCESS

$$
\begin{array}{r}
{\scriptstyle 1\ 1\ \ 1} \\
6.34 \\
12.45 \\
14.06 \\
+\ \ \underline{2.43} \\
\underline{35.28}
\end{array}
$$

Steps in vertical addition:

- Set out with numbers clearly and correctly placed under columns.
- Add in vertical format moving from right to left.
- Record only single digits under each column and regroup or carry over when required.
- Record 'carry over' digits at top of column in clear notation and don't forget to include when adding.
- This process is repeated whenever required.

Vertical subtraction

HINTS

- When subtracting smaller numbers from larger numbers, the largest number is recorded on the top. Use vertical formations, move from right to left.
- Subtraction answers can be checked by applying the inverse operation of addition, i.e. add answer to number subtracted, original number subtracted from should be found.

PROCESS

e.g.
$$
\begin{array}{r}
\overset{6}{5}\,\overset{15}{\not{7}}\,\overset{17}{\not{6}}\,\not{7} \\
-\,4\,3\,7\,8 \\
\hline
1\,3\,8\,9
\end{array}
$$

Steps:

- Set out with numbers clearly and correctly placed under columns.
- Work from the top number and say:
  — 7 take away 8 can't be done.
  — Regroup 1 ten from the existing 6 tens thus leaving 5 tens and making 17 in the ones column (show your workings).
  — 17 take away 8 leaves 9.
  — Record 9 under the ones column.
  — 5 take away 7 can't be done.
  — Regroup 1 from the next column thus leaving 6 and making the 5 into 15 (show your workings).
  — 15 take away 7 leaves 8.
  — Record 8 under the tens column.

— 6 take away 3 leaves 3.
— Record 3 under the hundreds column.
— 5 take away 4 leaves 1.
— Record 1 under the thousands column.

The answer is 1389.

When **subtracting with decimals**, follow the same format but ensure the 'PUP' rule is followed.

Multiplication

HINTS

- When multiplying using vertical formation move from right to left. ←
- When carrying or regrouping in multiplication, the carried number is added *after* the multiplication in each column has been done.
- *When multiplying by 10, 100, 1000 simply add the number of zeros of the base 10 number onto the end of the whole number, e.g. 23 × 1000 = 23 000.*

MULTIPLYING BY ONE-DIGIT NUMBER

PROCESS

e.g.
$$\begin{array}{r} {}^{1} \\ 342 \\ \times\ 4 \\ \hline 1368 \end{array}$$

Steps:
- 4 times 2 is 8.
  Record 8 under the ones column.
- 4 times 4 is 16.
  Record 6 under the tens column and regroup or carry over the 1 into the hundreds column. Record the 1 above the 3 and *ADD* after the next step.
- 4 times 3 is 12, plus the 1 regrouped = 13.
  Record 13, as there are no more numbers to multiply.

The answer is 1368.

MULTIPLYING BY TWO-DIGIT NUMBERS

PROCESS

e.g.
$$\begin{array}{r} \overset{1}{4142} \\ \times\ 14 \\ \hline 16\ 568 \\ +\ 41\ 420 \\ \hline 57\ 988 \end{array}$$

Steps:
- Follow the same steps as per multiplication by one digit.
  ↓
- Multiply the top line by 4 to get 16 568.
- Record zero in units column on next line (multiplying by tens).
- Multiply the top line by 1 as done previously to get 41 420.
- The two answers are then added together to achieve the final answer: 57 988.

The process of including zeros on each line in vertical multiplication equates to the number you are multiplying by.

i.e. Multiplying by

1 digit	→	no zero
2 digits	→	0 (tens)
3 digits	→	00 (hundreds)
4 digits	→	000 (thousands)

MULTIPLYING WITH DECIMALS

HINTS

• When multiplying decimals by 10, 100, 1000 and so on, move the decimal point to the right in accordance with the same number of zeros.

e.g.

13.254 × 10 = 132.54 (move one place because 10 has one zero)

13.254 × 100 = 1325.4 (move two places because 100 has two zeros)

MULTIPLYING DECIMALS BY A WHOLE NUMBER

PROCESS

e.g.
$$\begin{array}{r} 25.60 \\ \times\ \ \downarrow 15 \end{array}$$

Do as regular multiplication with two-digit number.

Place decimal point as indicated (PUP).

MULTIPLYING DECIMALS BY DECIMALS

PROCESS

e.g.   35.13 × 5.2

Ignore decimal point and multiply as whole numbers.

(Do not erase decimal points as they are important.)

Multiply as per multiplication by two or more digits.

```
    3 513
  ×   52
    7 026
  175 650
  182 676
```

When answer is gained count the number of digits after the decimal places in both original numbers. This will indicate where to put your decimal point in the answer.

i.e. 35.13 = two digits
     5.2 = one digit
         ↓

gives a total of three digits

Place the decimal point three digits from the right in answer.
= 182.676

Division
DIVIDING BY ONE DIGIT (SHORT DIVISION)
HINTS
The order of division is important.

Complete division equations from left to right.
→

PROCESS

e.g.
```
       22 42
    3)67¹26
```

Steps:
- Say: 6726 divided by 3; or 3 divided into 6726.
- Record using

  quotient
  divisor $\overline{)}$ dividend

- 3 divided into 6 = 2.
- Record answer '2' above 6.
- 3 divided into 7 = 2 remainder 1.
- Record '2' above 7 and regroup remaining 1 to make 12.
- 3 divided into 12 = 4.
- Record 4 above 12.
- 3 divided into 6 = 2.
- Record 2 above the 6.

The answer is 2242.

DIVIDING BY TWO DIGITS (LONG DIVISION)

HINTS

- Applied when dividing by a two-digit number. This follows the same process as short division but the regrouping process is written below the dividend.

PROCESS

$$
\begin{array}{r}
183 \text{ r } 23 \\
25\overline{)4598} \\
-25\downarrow \\
\hline
209 \\
-200\downarrow \\
\hline
98 \\
-75 \\
\hline
23
\end{array}
$$

e.g.

Steps:

- Say 4598 divided by 25; or 25 divided into 4598.
- Record as per short division and move from left to right.
- 25 divided into 45 = 1.
- Record 1 above 5.
- Subtract ($1 \times 25 = 25$) from 45 = 20.
- Bring down the next digit (9).
- 25 divided into 209 = 8.
- Record 8 above the 9.
- Subtract ($8 \times 25 = 200$) from 209 = 9.
- Bring down the next digit (8).
- 25 divided into 98 = 3.
- Record 3 above the 8.
- Subtract ($3 \times 25 = 75$) from 98 = 23.
- There are no more digits to bring down and 25 cannot divide into 23, so 23 becomes a remainder, which is recorded as r 23.

DIVISION WITH DECIMALS

HINTS

- When dividing by any number with a base 10, e.g. 100, 1000, count the number of zeros in the digit and move the decimal point that number to the left.

  e.g. $1843.6 \div 10 = 184.36$ (move one place because 10 has one zero)

  $1843.6 \div 100 = 18.436$ (move two places because 100 has two zeros)

DECIMAL DIVIDED BY WHOLE NUMBER

PROCESS

- Follow same steps for standard division.
- Record decimal point in line with dividend.

$$
\begin{array}{r}
7.03 \\
5\overline{)35.15}
\end{array}
$$

e.g.

DECIMALS DIVIDED BY DECIMALS

PROCESS

- Change the divisor into a whole number.
- Move the decimal point to the right in both numbers (divisor and dividend) by the same number of places.
- Follow the same steps for standard division,
  e.g. $25.35 \div 0.5$
- We need to move one decimal place to make the divisor into a whole number, so move one decimal place on dividend as well.

e.g. $253.5 \div 5$
$$\downarrow$$
$$
\begin{array}{r}
50.7 \\
5\overline{)253.5}
\end{array}
$$

■ WORKING WITH FRACTIONS

A patient is required to have an intravenous infusion of normal saline fluid of 1000 mL over a period of 8 hours. The drop factor is 20 mL. The nurse should set out the calculation as follows:

$$\frac{1000 \times 20}{8 \times 60}$$

The nurse needs to know how to work with fractions to solve problems such as this.

Fraction	A fraction refers to parts of a whole.
Numerator	Refers to the number above the (line) and represents the number of fractional parts.
Denominator	Refers to the number below the line and indicates how many equal fractional parts the whole has been divided into.
Proper fraction	A fraction with the numerator less than the denominator.
Improper fraction	A fraction with the numerator greater than the denominator.
Equivalent fractions	Fractions that equate to the same amount.
	They can be cancelled out to the same common fraction, e.g. $\frac{5}{10}$ and $\frac{4}{8}$ can be simplified to $\frac{1}{2}$
Lowest common denominator (LCD)	The LCD is the lowest common multiple of the denominators in two or more fractions, e.g. the LCD of $\frac{3}{5}$ and $\frac{1}{3}$ is 15 because 15 is the lowest number into which 3 and 5 divide exactly. LCDs are used when adding and subtracting fractions.
Mixed	A whole number and a fraction, e.g. $2\frac{1}{2}$

Decimals	Decimals are fractions that have denominators with powers of 10, e.g. 10, 100, 1000 etc. They are recorded using digits from $0 \rightarrow 9$. Decimals use a dot or point which separates the decimal fraction from the whole number (see place value chart above). Decimal notation is also used to show very large numbers, e.g. 7.2M = 7 200 000 (seven million and two hundred thousand).
Decimal fraction	A fraction that has been written as a decimal, e.g. $\frac{2}{10} \rightarrow 0.2$
Recurring decimal	A decimal fraction that has a repeating pattern, e.g. $\frac{1}{3} \rightarrow 0.33333$

Remember

Numerator is the number on the top.

Denominator is the number on the bottom. $\frac{6}{12}$

Converting fractions to decimals

The numerator is divided by the denominator.

e.g.

$$\frac{2}{3} = 2 \div 3 = 0.66$$

Converting decimals to fractions

Refer back to place value.

e.g.

$$0.7 = \frac{7}{10} \qquad 3.6 = 3\frac{6}{10}$$

Converting mixed to improper fractions	1. Multiply the whole number by the denominator. 2. Add on the numerator. 3. Place amount over the denominator. e.g. $2\frac{2}{3} \rightarrow 2 \times 3 = 6 \rightarrow 6 + 2 = 8 \rightarrow \frac{8}{3}$
Converting improper fractions to mixed fractions	1. Divide the numerator by the denominator. 2. Write the whole number. 3. Record any remainder over the denominator. e.g. $\frac{12}{5} \rightarrow 12 \div 5 = 2$ remainder $2 \rightarrow 2\frac{2}{5}$

Finding fractions of quantity	1. 'of' means to multiply.
	2. Whole numbers are written with 1 as the denominator, e.g. $12 = 12 = \frac{12}{1}$
	3. If working with mixed units, e.g. L and mL, hours and minutes, convert to same unit.
	e.g. Find $\frac{2}{3}$ of 20 (of means to multiply)
	$\rightarrow \frac{2}{3} \times \frac{20}{1}$ (20 is the same as $\frac{20}{1}$)
	$\rightarrow \dfrac{2 \times 20 = 40}{3 \times 1 = 3}$ (multiply the numerators)
	(multiply the denominators)
	$\rightarrow \frac{40}{3} = 13$ (convert improper fraction)
	remainder 1
	$\frac{2}{3}$ of $20 \approx 13.3$
Adding and subtracting fractions	**Adding and subtracting proper fractions with different denominators**
	1. Find the lowest common denominator (LCD).
	2. Change existing fractions to equivalent fractions using LCD.
	3. Add or subtract the numerator only.
	4. Change from improper to mixed and simplify if necessary.
	e.g. $\frac{5}{6} + \frac{2}{3} \rightarrow \frac{5}{6} + \frac{4}{6} = \frac{9}{6} \rightarrow 1\frac{3}{6} \rightarrow 1\frac{1}{2}$

Multiplying fractions	**Multiplying fractions**
	1. Change mixed fraction to improper fraction (cross cancelling can be done to simplify when multiplying).
	2. Multiply numerators.
	3. Multiply denominators.
	4. Change from improper to mixed and simplify if necessary.
	e.g. $1\frac{3}{5} \times 1\frac{2}{3} \rightarrow \frac{8}{5} \times \frac{5}{3} = \frac{40}{15} \rightarrow \frac{8}{3} \rightarrow 2\frac{2}{3}$
Dividing fractions	**Dividing proper fractions**
	1. Change divide ($\div$) into a multiplication ($\times$).
	2. Invert (turn upside down) the second fraction.
	3. Follow rules for multiplication of fractions.
	e.g. $\frac{5}{6} \div \frac{2}{3} \rightarrow \frac{5}{6} \times \frac{3}{2} = \frac{15}{12} \rightarrow 1\frac{3}{12} \rightarrow 1\frac{1}{4}$
	Dividing mixed fractions
	1. Change mixed fraction to improper fraction.
	2. Change divide into multiplication.
	3. Invert second fraction.
	4. Follow rules for multiplication of fractions.
	e.g. $2\frac{2}{3} \div 1\frac{1}{2} \rightarrow \frac{8}{3} \div \frac{3}{2} \rightarrow \frac{8}{3} \times \frac{2}{3} = \frac{16}{9} \rightarrow 1\frac{7}{9}$

■ PERCENTAGES

A percentage indicates number of parts in a hundred.

Nurses deal with percentages in clinical situations. For example, a patient may be ordered 15% of a particular drug in 120 mL solution of normal saline. Another example is that a patient may be assessed for burns in terms of percentage of the burn over the body. Calculations involving percentages may require the following methodology.

Finding the percentage of a quantity % **of**	e.g. Find 15% of 120 mL. There are three possible ways to do this. 1. Change percentage into fraction with **denominator of 100 × quantity**. e.g. 15% of 120 mL = $\frac{15}{100} \times \frac{120}{1}$ cross cancel $\rightarrow \frac{15}{10} \times \frac{12}{1} = \frac{180}{10} = 18$ mL 2. **Simplify percentage × quantity**. e.g. $\frac{15}{100} = \frac{3}{20} \times \frac{120}{1}$ cross cancel $\rightarrow \frac{3}{2} \times \frac{12}{1} = \frac{36}{2} = \frac{18}{1} = 18$ mL 3. Change percentage to **decimal form × quantity**. e.g. $0.15 \times 120 = 18$ mL
Finding quantity from a percentage % **=**	e.g. If 5% of total intake is 130 mL, what is the total intake required? 1. Find 1% of quantity by dividing quantity by percentage number: $130 \div 5 = 26$ 2. Multiply answer × 100% to get total amount: $26 \times 100 = 2600$ Total intake is 2600 mL.

To convert a percentage into a decimal: divide by 100.

e.g. 33% as a decimal is $33 \div 100 = 0.33$

To convert a percentage into a fraction: divide by 100.

e.g. 40% as a fraction is $\dfrac{40}{100}$

To convert a decimal to a percentage: multiply by 100.

e.g. 0.23 as a percentage is $0.23 \times 100 = 23\%$

To convert a fraction into a percentage: multiply by 100.

e.g. $\dfrac{2}{4}$ as a percentage is $\dfrac{2}{4} \times \dfrac{100}{1} = \dfrac{200}{4} = 50\%$

■ ROUNDING

If the digit to the right of the number is 5 or more, round up.

If the digit to the right of the number is less than 5, round down.

e.g. 2.185

Rounded to a whole number is 2

Rounded to one decimal place is 2.2

Rounded to two decimal places is 2.19

■ THE METRIC SYSTEM

The metric system is integral to nursing practice. It is fundamental for a nurse to understand this in order to perform safe drug calculations.

Gram (g)	Unit of mass
Litre (L)	Unit of volume
Metre (m)	Unit of length
Mole (mol)	Unit of substance

Measurement prefixes

PREFIX	ABBREVIATION	PLACE VALUE
Mega	M	1 000 000
Kilo	k	1 000
Hecto	h	100
Deka (deca)	da	10
Deci	d	0.1
Centi	c	0.01
Milli	m	0.001
Micro	mc or μ	0.000 001
Nano	n	0.000 000 001
Pico	p	0.000 000 000 001

Metric equivalents

Volume	
1 litre (L)	= 1000 millilitres (mL)
	= 1000 cc (cubic centimetres)
Mass	
1 kilogram (kg)	= 1000 grams (g)
1 gram (g)	= 1000 milligrams (mg)
1 milligram (mg)	= 1000 micrograms (mcg)
	or (μg)
Length	
1 kilometre (km)	= 1000 metres (m)
1 metre (m)	= 100 centimetres (cm)
1 centimetre (cm)	= 10 millimetres (mm)
Examples of equivalents	
0.2 kilograms	= 200 grams
0.2 grams	= 200 milligrams
0.2 milligrams	= 200 micrograms
0.2 litres	= 200 millilitres

Converting measuring units

Parts of a calculation may also require a nurse to convert measurements.

Converting is relatively easy if you know the metric equivalents.

To change milligrams to grams divide by 1000, moving the decimal point three places to the left.

1000 mg = 1 g
450 mg = 0.45 g

To convert litres to millilitres multiply by 1000 or move the decimal point three places to the right

$$1 \text{ L} = 1000 \text{ mL}$$
$$0.45 \text{ L} = 450 \text{ mL}$$

Note *Never confuse mL with units when working out dosages for drugs such as insulin.*
Absolute caution must be taken when administering drugs that are ordered in units.
Appropriate syringes must be used to determine that measurement is accurate.

Although the metric system is used in the UK, on occasion nurses may be asked by patients what the measurement means in the imperial system. For example, when an infant is born the parents may ask how much the child weighs in pounds.

The following table shows conversions.

Metric and imperial conversions

IMPERIAL	METRIC
1 stone	= 6.4 kg
1 pound	= 0.5 kg
1 foot	= 30.5 cm
1 inch	= 2.5 cm

WEIGHT CONVERSION FACTORS

Stones to kilograms:	× 6.3503
Pounds to kilograms:	× 0.4536
Kilograms to stones:	× 0.1575
Kilograms to pounds:	× 2.2046

HEIGHT CONVERSION FACTORS

Feet to centimetres:	× 30.48
Inches to centimetres:	× 2.54
Centimetres to feet:	× 0.0328
Centimetres to inches:	× 0.3937

Some handy tables involving measurement

■ INTRAVENOUS FLUID REQUIREMENTS

When measuring a child's weight it is important to consider whether their weight is average or below average, and what this might mean for the drug dosage they have been prescribed.

Average weights

Age In years	Term	3 mth	6 mth	1 yr	2 yr	4 yr
Weight in kg	3.5	6	8	10	13	15
Age In years	6 yr	8 yr	10 yr	12 yr	14 yr	17 yr+
Weight in kg	20	25	30	40	50	70

Reference / Adapted from Marks, M., Munro, J. and Paxton, G. (eds.) (2005) *Paediatric Handbook*, 7th edn. Brisbane, Australia: Blackwell Publishing. Reproduced with permission of Wiley-Blackwell Publishing Ltd.

Handy fluid measurements to know

1 cup	= 250 mL
$\frac{1}{4}$ cup	= 60 mL
$\frac{1}{2}$ cup	= 125 mL
$\frac{1}{4}$ teaspoon	= 1.25 mL
$\frac{1}{2}$ teaspoon	= 2.5 mL
1 teaspoon	= 5 mL
1 tablespoon	= 20 mL

Note *Variations may exist pending types of equipment that are used in organisations.*

Body mass index (BMI)

Calculation of body mass index (BMI) is achieved by using the formula:

weight (kg) / [height (m)]^2

Calculation:

[weight (kg) / height (m) $\times$ height (m)]

The formula for BMI is weight in kilograms divided by height in metres squared. As height is commonly measured in centimetres, divide height in centimetres by 100 to obtain height in metres.

e.g. Height = 165 cm (1.65 m), Weight = 68 kg
Calculation: $68 \div (1.65)^2 = 24.98$

BMI	
< 20	Underweight
20–25	Acceptable
25–30	Overweight
30–40	Obese
> 40	Morbidly obese

Reference / Adapted from Lapham, R. and Agar, H. (2003) *Drug Calculations for Nurses: A Step by Step Approach*, London: Hodder Arnold, p. 213. Reproduced by permission of Hodder Education.

■ RULE OF NINES

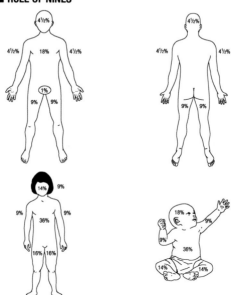

Above is the formula for estimating the percentage of burns on an adult body surface area.

This is modified below for infants and children.

Reference / Adapted from Harris, P., Nagy, S. and Vardaxis, N. (2006) *Mosby's Dictionary of Medicine, Nursing and Health Professions*, 7th edn. St. Louis, Missouri: Mosby, p. 1527. Reproduced with permission of Elsevier.

Formulas used in nursing

■ CALCULATING DOSAGE USING A FORMULA

Many formulas can be used to calculate medication dosages.

When preparing solids or liquid forms the following basic formulas can be applied.

Tablets

$$\frac{\text{Strength required}}{\text{Strength in stock}} \times \frac{\text{Volume}}{1} = \text{amount to be administered}$$

Mixtures and injectables

$$\frac{\text{Strength required}}{\text{Strength in stock}} \times \frac{\text{Volume}}{1} \qquad \frac{\text{SR}}{\text{SS}} \times \text{Volume}$$

$$\frac{\text{Dose prescribed}}{\text{Dose in stock}} \times \frac{\text{Volume}}{1} \qquad \frac{\text{DP}}{\text{DS}} \times \text{Volume}$$

However it is stated, it all says the same thing:

$$\frac{\text{What you want}}{\text{What you have}} \times \frac{\text{Volume}}{1}$$

$$\frac{\text{Want}}{\text{Got}} \times \frac{\text{Volume}}{1}$$

Intravenous fluids—drops/minute (dpm)

$$\frac{\text{Volume(mL)} \times \textbf{Drop factor (drops/mL)}^*}{\text{Time (hours)} \times 60 \text{ (minutes)}}$$

*CHECK the information on the giving set packaging for confirmation of drop factor.

Intravenous drip rates—calculating how many hours the intravenous infusion will run

$$\frac{\text{Volume (mL)}}{\text{Rate (mL/hour)}} = \text{Time (hours)}$$

When undertaking medication administration calculations REMEMBER:

- Read the medication order/prescription thoroughly.
- Read the medication drug packaging.
- Sort out what the dosage problem is.
- Use your mathematical manipulation skills to convert measuring units if necessary.
- Apply the appropriate formula and calculate.
- Reflect on the dosage:
  Is this reasonable?
  Is this within normal range?
  What are the consequences to the patient with this dosage?
- Check the dosage and your calculations with a second person.

Applying drug calculations using formulas

■ CALCULATING ORAL MEDICATIONS

Example simple oral medication

Date	Drug (use generic name) print	
11/09/11	Drug Antihypertensive	
Route	**Dose and frequency**	
PO	30 mg BD	
Pharmacy	**Dr Signature**	
		Print name
	V. Derry	Dr V.R. Derry
	Instructions	**Discharge supply**

The drug Antihypertensive is available as either 10 mg or 20 mg per tablet.

The formula may be stated as:

$$\frac{\text{Strength required}}{\text{Strength in stock}} \times \frac{\text{Volume}}{1}$$

$$\frac{\text{SR}}{\text{SS}} \times \frac{\text{Volume}}{1}$$

$$\frac{30 \text{ mg}}{20 \text{ mg}} \times \frac{1 \text{ tablet}}{1} = 30 \div 20 = 1.5 \text{ tablets}$$

or

$$\frac{30 \text{ mg}}{10 \text{ mg}} \times \frac{1 \text{ tablet}}{1} = 3 \text{ tablets}$$

Example complex oral medication based on body weight: mg/kg

Date	Drug (use generic name) print	
11/09/2011	Drug Antipyretic (children)	
Route	**Dose and frequency**	
PO	15 mg/kg 4 hourly up to 4 times/day	
Pharmacy	**Dr Signature**	
		Print name
	V. Derry	Dr V.R. Derry
	Instructions Child weighs 20 kg	**Discharge supply**

The drug Antipyretic (children) is available as 120 mg/5 mL. Therefore strength required:

$$15 \text{ mg} \times 20 \text{ kg} = 300 \text{ mg}$$

$$\frac{SR}{SS} \times \frac{Volume}{1}$$

$$\frac{300 \text{ mg}}{120 \text{ mg}} \times \frac{5 \text{ mL}}{1} = \text{mL to be administered}$$

Simplify the fraction: divide numerator and denominator by 20.

$$\frac{15}{6} \times \frac{5}{1}$$

Multiply the numerators:

$$\frac{75}{6}$$

$$75 \div 6 = 12.5 \text{ mL}$$

■ CALCULATING PARENTERAL MEDICATIONS

Calculating IV drug volumes

Date	Drug (use generic name) print	
11/09/2011	Drug Anticholinergic	
Route	**Dose and frequency**	
IVI	600 mcg PRN	
Pharmacy	**Dr Signature**	**Print name**
	V. Derry	Dr V.R. Derry
	Instructions	**Discharge supply**

The drug Anticholinergic is available as 1 mg/10 mL.

Therefore strength stock is 100 mcg/1 mL.

$$\frac{SR}{SS} \times \frac{Volume}{1}$$

$$\frac{600 \text{ mcg}}{100 \text{ mcg}} \times \frac{1 \text{ mL}}{1} = 600 \div 100 \times 1 = 6 \text{ mL}$$

Calculating intravenous rate—mL/hour

EXAMPLE 1

DATE/TIME	FLUID TYPE	DRUG (USE GENERIC NAME) ADDITIVE AND DOSE	TOTAL VOLUME (ML)	RATE	DR SIGNATURE PRINT NAME	START TIME
13/09/11 10.00	NaCl 0.9%	20 mmol KCl	1000 mL	6 h	*V. Derry* Dr V.R. Derry	06.00

Note *The giving set is 20 drops/mL.*

The formula is $\dfrac{Volume \text{ (mL)}}{Time \text{ (hours)}}$

$$\frac{1000 \text{ mL}}{6 \text{ hours}} = 166.6 \text{ mL/hour rounded up to 167 mL/hour}$$

EXAMPLE 2

DATE/TIME	FLUID TYPE	DRUG (USE GENERIC NAME) ADDITIVE AND DOSE	TOTAL VOLUME (ML)	RATE	DR SIGNATURE PRINT NAME	START TIME
13/09/11 10.00	NaCl 0.9%		100 mL	30 min	*V. Derry* Dr V.R. Derry	06.00

Note *The giving set is 20 drops/mL.*

The rate is 100 mL over 30 minutes. You first need to convert minutes to hours.

Either divide the required minutes by 60 (60 minutes in the hour):

$$\frac{30}{60} = 0.5$$

The formula is $\frac{\text{Volume (mL)}}{\text{Time (hours)}}$

$$\frac{100 \text{ mL}}{0.5 \text{ hour}} = 200 \text{ mL/hour}$$

Or convert the minutes to hours. As there are 2×30 minutes in the hour ($\frac{60}{30} = 2$),

$$\frac{100 \times 2}{30 \text{ minutes} \times 2} \text{ which is the same as } \frac{100 \times 2}{1 \text{ hour}}$$

$$= 200 \text{ mL/hour}$$

Intravenous drip rates—drops/minute (dpm)

The formula is $\dfrac{\text{Volume (mL)}}{\text{Time (hours)}} \times \dfrac{\text{Drop factor (drops/mL)}}{60 \text{ (minutes)}}$

EXAMPLE 1

DATE/TIME	FLUID TYPE	DRUG (USE GENERIC NAME) ADDITIVE AND DOSE	TOTAL VOLUME (ML)	RATE	DR SIGNATURE PRINT NAME	START TIME
13/09/11 10.00	NaCl 0.9%		1000 mL	1000 mL/ 6 h	*V. Derry* Dr V.R. Derry	06.00

Note The giving set is 20 drops/mL.

$$\frac{1000 \text{ (mL)}}{6 \text{ (hours)}} \times \frac{20 \text{ (drops/mL)}}{60 \text{ (minutes)}} = 55.55 \text{ drops/minute}$$
$$\text{round} = 56 \text{ dpm}$$

EXAMPLE 2

DATE/TIME	FLUID TYPE	DRUG (USE GENERIC NAME) ADDITIVE AND DOSE	TOTAL VOLUME (ML)	RATE	DR SIGNATURE PRINT NAME	START TIME
13/09/11 10.00	NaCl 0.9%		100 mL	100 mL/ 20 min	*V. Derry* Dr V.R. Derry	06.00

Note The giving set is 60 drops/mL.

$$\frac{100 \text{ (mL)}}{20 \text{ (minutes)}} \times \frac{60 \text{ (drops/mL)}}{60 \text{ (minutes)}} = 300 \text{ dpm}$$

Intravenous drip rates—calculating how many hours the IVT will run

The formula is $\dfrac{\text{Volume (mL)}}{\text{Rate (mL/hour)}} = \text{Time (hours)}$

EXAMPLE

1000 mL bag of fluid and pump set at 84 mL/hour.

$$\dfrac{1000 \text{ mL}}{84 \text{ mL/hour}} = 11.9 \text{ hours rounded to 12 hours}$$

Intravenous drip rates—converting dosages to mL/hour

DATE/TIME	FLUID TYPE	DRUG (USE GENERIC NAME) ADDITIVE AND DOSE	TOTAL VOLUME (ML)	RATE	DR SIGNATURE PRINT NAME	START TIME
13/09/11 05.00	5% Dextrose	Drug Analgesic 30 mg	30 mL	1 mL/h*	*V. Derry* Dr V.R. Derry	06.00

*1 mL/h =1 mg Analgesic/hour

Note The giving set is 20 drops/mL.

Calculate how many mL/hour to run the drip.

The drug Analgesic is available in 30 mg in 1 mL ampoule to be diluted in a total of 30 mL 5% Dextrose. So 1 mL of the drug Analgesic and 29 mL 5% Dextrose (total of 30 mL) is required.

Therefore the final concentration is 1 mL = 1 mg.

The IVT pump is to be set at 1 mL/hour. Or:

$$\frac{\text{Strength required}}{\text{Strength in stock}} \times \frac{\text{Volume}}{1}$$

$$\frac{1 \text{ mg/hour}}{30 \text{ mg}} \times \frac{30 \text{ mL}}{1} = 1 \text{ mL/hour}$$

Calculating medication dosage—mg/hour

DATE/TIME	FLUID TYPE	DRUG (USE GENERIC NAME) ADDITIVE AND DOSE	TOTAL VOLUME (ML)	RATE	DR SIGNATURE PRINT NAME	START TIME
13/09/11 05.00	5% Dextrose	Drug Diuretic 80 mg	40 mL	2–6 mL/h	*V. Derry* Dr V.R. Derry	06.00

Note The giving set is 20 drops/mL.

The formula is

$$\frac{\text{Strength required (mg/h)}}{\text{Strength in stock (mg)}} \times \frac{\text{Volume (mL)}}{1} = \text{mL/hour}$$

EXAMPLE

The drug Diuretic has been ordered at a rate of 2–6 mg/hour (intravenously) and is currently running at 3 mL/hour. How many mg/hour is the drip running at?

The drug Diuretic is available as 40 mg/4 mL.

8 mL (80 mg) of the drug Diuretic is added to 32 mL Dextrose 5% (total of 40 mL).

The final concentration is 2 mg in 1 mL of solution.

$$2 \text{ mg/mL} \times 3 \text{ mL/hr} = 6 \text{ mg/hour}$$

Or

$$\frac{??? \text{ mg/hour}}{80 \text{ mg}} \times \frac{40 \text{ mL}}{1} = 3 \text{ mL/hour}$$

$$= 6 \text{ mg/hour}$$

Calculating intravenous rate—mcg/minute

DATE/TIME	FLUID TYPE	DRUG (USE GENERIC NAME) ADDITIVE AND DOSE	VOLUME (ML)	RATE	DR SIGNATURE PRINT NAME	START TIME
13/09/11 05.00	5% Dextrose	Drug Vasopressor 6 mg	60 mL	2 mL/h	*V. Derry* Dr V.R. Derry	06.00

The formula is

$$\frac{\text{Dose (mcg)}}{\text{Volume (mL)}} \times \frac{\text{Rate (mL/hour)}}{60} = \text{mcg/min}$$

EXAMPLE

The drug Vasopressor has been ordered to run at 2 mL/hour. The drug Vasopressor is available as 1 mg/1 mL or 1000 mcg/1 mL.

6 mL (6 mg) of the drug Vasopressor is added to 54 mL 5% Dextrose (total of 60 mL). There are 6 mg in 60 mL and therefore 6000 mcg in 60 mL. Which is the same as

600 mcg in 6 mL. The final concentration is 1 mg for 10 mL of solution *or* 100 mcg/1 mL.

$$\frac{600 \ (\text{mcg})}{6 \ \text{mL}} \times \frac{2 \ (\text{mL/hour})}{60} = 3.3 \ \text{mcg/minute}$$

Calculating mcg/kg/minute

The formula is

$$\frac{\text{Dose (mcg)}}{\text{Volume (mL)}} \times \frac{\text{Rate (mL/hour)}}{60} \times \frac{1}{\text{Weight (kg)}}$$

EXAMPLE 1

DATE/TIME	FLUID TYPE	DRUG (USE GENERIC NAME) ADDITIVE AND DOSE	TOTAL VOLUME (ML)	RATE	DR SIGNATURE PRINT NAME	START TIME
13/09/11 05.00	5% Dextrose	Drug Inotrope 200 mg	100 mL	5 mL/h	*V. Derry* Dr V.R. Derry	06.00

The drug Inotrope has been ordered to run at 5 mL/hour. The drug Inotrope is available as 200 mg in 5 mL. The patient weighs 75 kg.

5 mL (200 mg) of the drug Inotrope is added to 95 mL 5% Dextrose (total of 100 mL).

The final concentration is 2 mg in 1 mL solution *or* 2000 mcg/1 mL.

$$\frac{200\,000 \ (\text{mcg})}{100 \ (\text{mL})} \times \frac{5 \ (\text{mL/hour})}{60} \times \frac{1}{75 \ (\text{kg})} = 2.2 \ \text{mcg/kg/min}$$

EXAMPLE 2

The formula given on page 50 can be rearranged to find the rate in mL/hour.

DATE/TIME	FLUID TYPE	DRUG (USE GENERIC NAME) ADDITIVE AND DOSE	TOTAL VOLUME (ML)	RATE	DR SIGNATURE PRINT NAME	START TIME
13/09/11 05.00	5% Dextrose	Drug Inotrope 200 mg	100 mL	5 mL/ kg/min	*V. Derry* Dr V.R. Derry	06.00

The drug Inotrope is available as 200 mg in 5 mL. The patient weighs 75 kg.

5 mL (200 mg) of the drug Inotrope is added to 95 mL 5% dextrose (total of 100 mL).

The final concentration is 2 mg in 1 mL solution *or* 2000 mcg/1mL.

$$\frac{200\,000 \text{ (mcg)}}{100 \text{ (mL)}} \times \frac{\text{Rate (mL/hour)}}{60} \times \frac{1}{75 \text{ (kg)}}$$

$$= 5 \text{ mcg/kg/min}$$

or

$$\frac{5 \text{ (mcg/kg/hour)}}{200\,000 \text{ (mL)}} \times 100 \text{ (mL)} \times 60 \times 75 \text{ (kg)}$$

$$= \text{Rate (mL/hour)} = 11.25 \text{ mL/hour}$$

Safe medication administration

■ CATEGORIES OF DRUGS

THREE CLASSES OF PRODUCT UNDER THE MEDICINES ACT 1968	
General Sales List Medicines (GSL)	Over the counter (OTC) drugs sold without the supervision of a pharmacist, e.g. Paracetamol – an analgesic
Pharmacy Medicines (P)	May only be sold under the supervision of a pharmacist, e.g. chlorphenamine – an antihistamine
Prescription Only Medicines (POM)	Only supplied in accordance with a prescription given by an appropriate practitioner. There are some exemptions, e.g. insulin.

MISUSE OF DRUGS REGULATIONS 1985 RELATES TO DRUGS THAT MAY CAUSE DEPENDENCE IF MISUSED.

These are referred to as 'Controlled Drugs' (CDs) and are divided into five schedules that govern supply, prescribing and record keeping.

Schedule 1	Not authorised for medical use, e.g. raw opium.
Schedule 2	Subject to full controlled-drug requirements and need a special register, e.g. morphine.
Schedule 3	Do not require a special register, e.g. buprenorphine.
Schedule 4	Subject to minimal control, e.g. diazepam.
Schedule 5	Drugs that are exempt from CD regulations due to strength, e.g. those containing less than 0.2% morphine.

■ WHAT MUST BE ON A PRESCRIPTION AND ADMINISTRATION RECORD

Must be written clearly in ink and indelible.

Every drug chart must include basic patient information:
- Patient's name and address
- Hospital number
- Patient's age and date of birth
- Patient's weight if dosage is related to weight
- Previous allergies

Details of the drug to be administered:
- The generic name, or brand name where appropriate, in capital letters
- The form the medication is to be in
- The route of administration
- The strength, dosage and frequency of administration
- The times to be taken using 24-hour clock
- Start and finish dates

Other details:
- The date
- The medical officer's printed name and signature

■ WHAT MAKES A PRESCRIPTION VALID

It should:

- Be written in ink and indelible
- Be signed and dated by the prescriber
- State the full name and address (unless in hospital) of the patient
- Give the date when the medication is to start
- Supply the printed generic name of the drug
- Specify the dose and frequency of administration

Reference / From Galbraith, A., Bullock, S., Manias, E., Hunt, B. and Richards, A. (2008) *Fundamentals of Pharmacology: An Applied Approach for Nursing and Health*, 2nd edn. Sydney: Pearson Education.

■ FREQUENCY AND TIMES OF MEDICATION ADMINISTRATION

Below is a guideline for administration times.

Morning	Mane	0800			
Night	Nocte			1800 or 2000	
Twice daily	BD	0800		2000	
Three times a day	TDS	0800	1400	2000	
Four times a day	QID	0600	1200	1800	2200

Reference / Australian Council for Safety and Quality in Health Care (2005) *National Inpatient Medication Chart Guidelines*. Sydney: Australian Council for Safety and Quality in Health Care. Copyright © Commonwealth of Australia. Reproduced by permission.

■ WHAT IS ON A MEDICATION LABEL

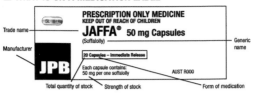

- Trade name of medication
- Generic name of medication
- Strength of stock
- Form of medication
- Manufacturer
- Quantity of stock

Note *A student should not take a telephone order. This is the responsibility of the Registered Nurse.*

■ COMMONLY USED AND UNDERSTOOD ABBREVIATIONS

Frequency

ABBREVIATION	MEANING
mane	morning
nocte	night
bd	twice daily
tds (tid)	three times a day
qid (qds)	four times a day
unit(s)	International Unit(s)

Dose

ABBREVIATION	MEANING
mL	millilitre
L	litre
g	gram
mg	milligram
mcg	microgram
unit(s)	International Unit(s)

Route

ABBREVIATION	MEANING
PO	by mouth
NG	nasogastric
SL	sublingual
IV	intravenous
IM	intramuscular
Subcut	subcutaneous
IT	intrathecal
PR	per rectum
PV	per vagina

ABBREVIATION	MEANING
Gutt	eye drop
Occ	eye ointment
Top	topical
MA	metered aerosol
Neb	nebulised/nebuliser

Reference / Australian Council for Safety and Quality in Health Care (2005) *National Impatient Medication Chart Guidelines*. Sydney: Australian Council for Safety and Quality in Health Care. Copyright © Commonwealth of Australia. Reproduced by permission.

■ OTHER ABBREVIATIONS

ABBREVIATION/SYMBOLS	MEANING
1/24	1 hourly
2/24	2 hourly
2/7	2 days
2/52	2 weeks
2/12	2 months
BSA	Body Surface Area
BMI	Body Mass Index

■ INTRAVENOUS FLUIDS—WHAT IS ON A FLUID ORDER

- Patient details
- Time in 24 hours
- Date
- Bag number
- Type of fluid
- Volume of fluid to be administered recorded in mL
- Duration of time fluid is to be administered
- Rate–speed at which fluid is to be administered
- Additives
- Medical officer's signature
- Time to be commenced
- Nurse's signature

■ ABBREVIATIONS FOR INTRAVENOUS FLUIDS

ABBREVIATION	FLUID TYPE
NaCl 0.9%; 0.9% saline; N/S; N/Saline	Normal saline/Isotonic saline
NaCl 0.45%; 0.45% saline	Half-strength saline
NaCl 3%; 3% saline	Hypertonic saline
5% Dex Dex 5% D_5W	5% dextrose (5% dextrose in water)

ABBREVIATION	FLUID TYPE
50% Dex $D_{50}W$	50% dextrose (50% dextrose in water)
Ringer's	Lactated Ringer's
4% and a 1/5 4% Dex/0.18% NaCl	4% dextrose in 1/5 saline
5% and NS 5% Dex/0.9% NaCl	5% dextrose in normal saline
FFP	Fresh frozen plasma
PC	Packed cells
Circle with dot in middle	Unit

■ INTRAVENOUS FLUIDS—DRIP RATES FOR GIVING SETS WHERE 20 DROPS = 1 ML

1000 ML	ML/HOUR	DROPS/MINUTE
q2h	500	167
q4h	250	83
q6h	167	56
q8h	125	42
q10h	100	33
q12h	83	28
q16h	63	21
q24h	42	14

■ THE PROCESS OF MEDICATION ADMINISTRATION
The 'Five Rights' and 'More'

Five rights
- Right patient
- Right drug
- Right dose
- Right time
- Right route

More than five rights
- Right to refuse
- Right person administering
- Right process followed
- Right documentation
- Right effect
- Right outcome

The NMC Standards for Medicines Management
Available in full from www.nmc-uk.org, the NMC Standards for Medicines Management replaced the Guidelines for the Administration of Medicines and are designed to reflect contemporary nursing practice. There are 26 Standards in 10 sections:

Section 1 – Methods of supplying and/or administration of medicines: Standards 1–3

Section 2 – Dispensing: Standards 4–5

Section 3 – Storage and Transportation: Standards 6–7

Section 4 – Standards for practice of administration of medicines: Standards 8–16

SECTION 4 is extremely relevant for Registered Nurses administering medicines, and so Standards 8–16 are outlined below.

Standard 8

- Be certain of the identity of the patient.
- Check the patient is not allergic to drug to be administered.
- Know the therapeutic uses, normal dosage, side effects, precautions and contraindications of the medicine (consult the British National Formulary (BNF) for this information).
- Be aware of the patient's plan of care.
- Check prescription and label on medicine is clearly written and unambiguous.
- Check expiry date of medicine (if it exists).
- Consider the dose, method of administration, route and timing.
- Administer or withhold according to patient's condition.
- Contact prescriber if reaction or medicine no longer suitable.
- Make a clear, accurate and immediate record of all medicines administered, withheld or refused by the patient and make sure your signature is clear.
- If medicine not given, the reason must be recorded.

- A Registered Nurse may administer with a single signature except for Controlled Drugs (CD) where a secondary signature is required from another registered health professional or a student nurse in most instances.
- The secondary signatory should witness the whole administration procedure for the CD.
- When supervising a student in medicine administration you must clearly countersign the signature of the student.

Standard 9: The registrant is responsible for assessment of patients who are self-administering.

Standard 10: Ensure medication administered by parents/carers to children has been taken.

Standard 11: In exceptional circumstances where medication has been **previously** prescribed but where a change in dose is needed, the use of fax, text message or e-mail may be considered.

Standard 12: Ensure patient confidentiality and accurate documentation regarding any text received.

Standard 13: A registrant may titrate dose according to patient response when a range of doses have been prescribed.

Standard 14: Do not prepare substances for injection in advance or administer from a syringe drawn up by another practitioner not in your presence.

Standard 15: Never administer any medication not prescribed, or acquired over the internet without a valid prescription.

Standard 16: Assess the patient's suitability and understanding of how to use any compliance aid safely.

Reference / Adapted from Nursing and Midwifery Council (2007) *Nursing and Midwifery Council Standards for Medicines Management*. London: NMC. Reproduced with permission.

Medication administration is more than just the five rights—it is about ensuring patient needs are met, that medicines have the desired effect and that safe outcomes result.

Three checks

1. Check the label when getting the drug from storage.
2. Check the drug label with the drug order.
3. Recheck the drug order and drug after dispensing but prior to administering.

■ MEDICATION ADMINISTRATION GUIDELINES FOR STUDENTS

- If you are to administer medication, assess that you are permitted to proceed.
- Always seek direct and personal supervision from a Registered Nurse.
- Do not administer medications without direct supervision.
- Assess what medication is needed.
- Use the BNF to understand action/interactions/side effects/doses/contraindication/route.
- Assess that the medication order is complete and valid.
- Check how the medication is to be administered.
- Gather correct equipment.
- Check the medication label.
- Check the expiry date.
- Calculate the drug dose and check this with the Registered Nurse.
- Prepare medication correctly.
- Use standard precautions.

- Follow five rights and more:
  — Right patient—check name, ID band, ask patient to state their name
  — Right drug—check medication order/drug
  — Right dose—check medication order/check BNF/check calculation
  — Right time—check medication order (24 hours)
  — Right route—check medication order and BNF
  — Right to refuse—check that the patient is willing
  — Right person administering—check that supervision is direct
  — Right process followed—check that all steps have been followed
- Do the three checks.
- Check allergies.
- At time of administration:
  — Check supervision is still apparent.
  — Confirm no allergies.
  — Check for contraindications for the patient receiving medication.
  — Prepare the patient—educate.
  — Administer medication and stay with patient.
- Right documentation—sign medication chart with the Registered Nurse and include the time of administration.
- Evaluate:
  — Right effect—check the patient to ensure effect and monitor.
  — Right outcome—check that the process has been correct.

Reference / Adapted from Glaister, K. (1997) *Medication Mathematics*, Melbourne: Macmillan Education Australia, pp. 56–7.

■ PREVENTING ERRORS

Tips for all medications

- Direct supervision from a Registered Nurse for students.
- Never give medications if you cannot read the medication chart.
- Do not give medication if elements on the order are missing.
- If in doubt, do not administer—seek advice.
- Always question large doses.
- Always double-check medication calculations.
- Check decimal points.
- Know measurements.
- Know the difference between units and mL.
- Never administer anything that you have not prepared yourself.
- Never leave medications beside a patient's bed.
- Always perform the five rights and more.
- Always conduct the three checks.

Tips for oral medications

- Measure oral liquids at eye level on a flat surface.
- Do not crush enteric-coated medications.
- When breaking scored medications use the appropriate device.
- When handling medications use standard precautions.
- Check that patient can swallow.
- Do not give if: the patient is sedated, has no gag reflex, no swallowing reflex or is vomiting.
- Sit patient up.
- Check that fluid is available to allow patient to swallow medications.
- Consider whether patient is on a fluid balance chart and record intake with medications.
- Stay with patient until medication has been swallowed.

Tips for injectable medications

- Check with two nurses.
- Have direct supervision.
- Check calculations.
- Take drug ampoule to bedside—allows for correct checking preadministration.
- Know the landmarks.
- Use correct needle and syringe.
- Never recap needle.
- Use standard precautions.
- Dispose of needle/syringe appropriately.

The 12 'knows' of safety

- Know that students need direct supervision.
- Know that this takes concentration.
- Know how to do your calculations.
- Know your mathematical conversions.
- Know the legalities surrounding your administering.
- Know the drugs—use the BNF.
- Know to listen to the patient.
- Know what makes a valid medication order.
- Know that there are more than five rights.
- Know the three checks.
- Know to follow manufacturer's instructions.
- Know to say no to: administering medication that someone else has prepared; administering without supervision.

Considerations for the paediatric patient

- Always have direct supervision from a Registered Nurse as a student.
- Double-check order.
- Question large doses.
- Check drug dosages with child's weight.
- Dosage determined, i.e. mg/kg, on ideal body weight. Take precaution with obese children.
- Check drug in paediatric BNF
- Gain child/caregiver's cooperation prior to administration.
- Never forcibly restrain a child.
- Position effectively.
- Never leave medications with child/caregiver.
- If child spits medication out or refuses, notify medical officer.

Tips for shift change over checks with medications and intravenous infusions

Students should perform the following checks with the Registered Nurse:

- Check medication chart:
  - have all medications been given and signed for on previous shift at the correct time?
  - what medications are due for the next shift?
- With intravenous infusions, check:
  - is the solution correct against the fluid orders?
  - is the solution infusing at the correct rate? Is the equipment set correctly?
  - if additives are infusing, are they correct?
  - are the lines correct?
  - is the patient's infusion site stable and without signs of phlebitis or infiltration into tissues?
  - has the fluid been hanging for less than 24 hours?
  - is the fluid balance chart up-to-date?

Shift roster

DAY	DATE	SHIFT
MONDAY		
TUESDAY		
WEDNESDAY		
THURSDAY		
FRIDAY		
SATURDAY		
SUNDAY		